STRETCHING FOR RUNNING

Christopher M. Norris

A&C BLACK, LONDON

Note Whilst every effort has been made to ensure the content of this book is as technically accurate as possible, neither the author nor the publishers can accept responsibility for any injury or loss sustained as a result of the use of this material.

First published in 2008 by
A & C Black Publishers Ltd
38 Soho Square
London W1D 3HB
www.acblack.com

© 2008 Christopher M. Norris

ISBN 978 14081 0694 5

A CIP catalogue record for this book is available from the British Library.

This book is produced using paper from wood grown in managed, sustainable forests. It is natural, renewable and recyclable. The logging and manufacturing processes conform to the environmental regulations of the country of origin.

Typeset in Din Light by Palimpsest Book Production Limited, Grangemouth, Stirlingshire

Cover image © Corbis
Inside photography © Grant Pritchard, except pages 2, 6, 60, 80, 90
© Shutterstock
Illustrations © Jeff Edwards

Printed and bound in China by South China Printing Co.

CONTENTS

Acknowledgements

My thanks go to Susie Gale, Victoria Jones, Jean Nadin, Madge Slater and Suzanne Hattersley, who modelled for the exercises.

In this case, you can use a warm-up to remind yourself of the movement. You can do this with a couple of simple actions and then build up the complexity: walking before you run, as it were. This is extremely important when you increase your running pace and begin sprint training, hill work, and simple running drills.

. . . and the bad

The idea of a warm-up is to prepare you for exercise. It should help you to perform the exercises better, and reduce the chances of injury. However, in some instances a warm-up can be detrimental.

Damage often occurs when extreme stretching is used as part of a warm-up. This is because, after extreme stretching, your muscles are tired and aching, and so you are more likely to be injured if, for example, you make a sudden, powerful movement. If your muscles are fatigued, you will also not be able to perform as well in a sport which involves heavy muscle work – if you were to do a short maximum sprint, for example. Stretching your leg muscles until they really ache will mean that you can't sprint as fast.

This is really common sense, but it is important to differentiate between the two types of stretching – maintenance and developmental – which we will cover below.

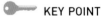 **KEY POINT**

A warm-up should make you sweat lightly, and rehearse the actions you are about to use in the sport.

Practical warm-up

So, how do we warm up? Well, a good warm-up should:
- take your joints and muscles through their normal degree of movement (range of motion);

- increase your pulse enough to make you sweat very lightly.

If you miss out some joints, or don't sweat at all, your warm-up is not intense enough (too easy), but if you sweat profusely or end up with aching muscles your warm-up is too intense (too hard).

Let's take a brief look at typical warm-ups before running and also before a stretching routine.

Before running or other sports

If you are simply going for a jog and you exercise regularly, you should begin by walking for 200m before you jog. This is fine, as a jog is low intensity for you. However, you will still need to stretch all your muscles – even your upper body and trunk – because although low intensity, a jog can still place stress on the shoulders and upper spine, especially if you are holding yourself tightly in these areas.

The situation is different if you are using running drills as part of your training for another sport (football or hockey, for example). You will need a more thorough warm-up before running drills, as this exercise is of a greater intensity than jogging. In this case jogging will actually form part of your warm-up.

In a gym, you can use CV (cardiovascular) machines such as the bike, treadmill, rower or cross-trainer. If using the treadmill, begin with a slow walk, building up to a brisk pace, and then raise the incline so you are marching uphill. After three or four minutes of this put the treadmill flat and start jogging. A 5–10 minute jog is sufficient to warm up your leg muscles and heart. Remember, however, that the treadmill does not work your arms substantially.

The bike works your arms even less, unless you use specific 'spin' exercises for the arms. Again, begin slowly and progress over a 5–10 minute period. The rower and cross-trainer are really better machines for a warm-up, because they give you a whole body effect. Because of this you may find that you sweat more quickly.

This 5–10 minute session takes care of the circulatory and body tissue elements of your warm-up. To warm up psychologically you will need to use movement rehearsal, and this is best done by performing the first set of any exercise at a lower intensity:

- With running drills, walk through the first drill to rehearse it, then progress to a slow jog through that drill and finally using the drill at full intensity.
- Before sprinting, again walk, jog and run, but also rehearse the arm action, slowly at first and then more quickly, using an exaggerated arm swing action.

In a maximum sprint you are not just using the same muscles more quickly – the action is different altogether. To sprint maximally you are stretching your muscles (especially the hamstrings on the back of your thigh, and your hip and quadriceps muscles at the front) and then allowing them to recoil like giant elastic bands. This is why stretching is vital for any sportsman or woman who uses sprinting in their sport. The springier your muscles are the faster you will sprint – and that will get you to the line before your opponent!

Before stretching
In the case of a stretching routine you would aim to warm up by moving 50–60 per cent of your motion range to begin with; then rest and increase this range to 80–90 per cent for the second set. Only stretch fully (100–110 per cent) when you are sure that you are completely warm. Remember, however, that you do not necessarily need to stretch to extreme levels with every session.

Stretching to warm up

When you are warming up using stretching, you should take your joint through its near maximum comfortable range, but no further (don't push it!). This is known as maintenance stretching: it is still stretching, of course, because if you have been sitting at your office desk all day, your muscles are stiff. You then need to stretch to your full range to get rid of the stiffness and lengthen your body tissues to their full, comfortable level. When you were sitting at work, you may have used only 20 per cent of your potential stretch; with maintenance stretching you can use 60–70 per cent.

Intensive (also known as developmental) stretching takes this range further: you move to 100 per cent of your range and then try to increase from this (105–110 per cent). Now you are actually trying to make your tissues more flexible that they have been before. *The golden rule is not to use intensive stretching before sport or as part of a warm-up.* Instead, you should warm up in order to stretch.

Putting stretches in a warm-up is fine providing you are using lower levels of stretching – perhaps 50–60 per cent of your movement range. Any more is counterproductive, as it will leave you sore and so affect your performance.

 KEY POINT

Make sure you are warm before you stretch. Don't use intensive stretching as part of a warm-up.

Checking your flexibility

Before you stretch it is helpful to record your current level of flexibility – how far you can actually stretch now. Why? Because this will be your baseline, the starting point against which you can measure your progress. If you don't know how flexible you were to begin with, you will often fail to see any progress in your stretching, because that progress will actually be quite slow. If you have nothing to measure progress against, it is easy to lose heart and become demotivated.

The other important reason to measure your flexibility is to find out whether your physique is balanced. Muscle imbalance is common, and occurs when some of your muscles are tight and when others are quite flexible. This is often brought about either by your job or by sport. In your job, if you sit hunched over a desk, you can easily become round-shouldered. This is a good example of muscle imbalance – your chest muscles are often tight, but your upper back muscles in contrast may be lax and too flexible. If you simply stretch all your muscles, you will certainly become more flexible, but your physique will still be imbalanced.

The chart on pages 14–18 shows some simple tests, which you can use to measure and record your current flexibility. You'll notice that this includes trunk and arms as well as legs: this is because, although the legs are used mostly in running, runners often suffer pain and stiffness around the shoulders and trunk, which we can target with stretching.

Following a warm-up, you should perform each of these tests, holding the fully stretched position for 10 seconds. Pull into the position slowly, with no bouncing movements. Measure your scores, and record them on the chart (make a photocopy if you do not want to mark your book). Your measurement will give you a score of same as, less than or more than the average, and you may find that this varies between exercises. Some may be poor, some good, and this shows that muscle imbalance is present.

The score is for your guidance only – your individual measurement is actually more important as it represents your baseline measure, the one which you will be comparing against. You can retest your flexibility using this chart every week throughout the stretching programme to monitor your progress.

Testing your flexibility

Tick the box that corresponds to your movement range, following the guidelines given for each test. Recheck each week.

- Remember to warm up first.
- Hold each stretch for three seconds before measuring.
- Do not bounce into the movement.
- Average values vary with body size and type.

Test	Less	Average	More
Keep your straight leg on the floor and pull your bent knee towards your chest	knee more than 15 cm from ribcage	knee 10–15 cm from ribcage	knee to ribcage
Place the soles of your feet together and press your knees downwards towards the floor	more than 15 cm from floor	15 cm from floor	less than 15 cm from floor
Keep your knees locked and reach forwards towards your toes	more than 15 cm from toes	10–15 cm from toes	touching toes

Test	Less	Average	More
Bend your lower leg up to your chest and hold still; lower your top leg towards the ground	above horizontal	horizontal	below horizontal
Stand 0.5 m from a wall. Lean forwards, keeping your feet flat on the floor and knees locked	more than 60°	60°	less than 60°
Keep your forehead and chest on the ground and lift your arms upwards	less than 15 cm	15–20 cm	more than 20 cm
Reach behind your back and try to grip the fingers of the opposite hand	fingers more than 15 cm apart	fingers 10–15 cm apart	fingers touching

Test	Less	Average	More
 Keep your arms straight and try to cross them over as far as possible	cross at wrist	cross at elbow	cross at upper arm
 Keep your foot flat on a stool and press your knee towards the wall	more than 50°	40–50°	less than 40°
 Keep your knees together and bent to 90°. Allow your heels to drop downwards	less than 70°	70–90°	more than 90°
 Lock your arms flat out and measure the distance between the top of your pelvis and the floor	more than 15 cm	15–10 cm	less than 10 cm

Test	Less	Average	More
Keeping your arms flat on the floor, twist your trunk to allow your knees to lower towards the floor	more than 10 cm from floor	up to 10 cm	0 cm
Keep the small of your back against the chair back and flex your spine (not your hips) as much as possible	fingers to mid-shin	fingers to floor	hand flat to floor
Keeping your feet flat and knees locked, reach down the side of your leg without leaning forwards or backwards	fingers above knee	fingers to knee	fingers below knee
Keep both legs straight and flex one hip as far as possible	less than 90°	90°	more than 90°

Test	Less	Average	More
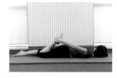 Push your legs apart while keeping the small of the back flat and your legs straight	less than 90° between legs	90°	more than 90°
 Keep your knees together and flex one knee as far as possible	heel more than 10 cm from buttock	heel 5–10 cm from buttock	heel to buttock
Keeping your knees and ankles together throughout, slowly sit back on your heels. Measure the distance between the top of the foot and the ground	more than 5 cm	up to 5 cm	flat

Types of stretching and how to use them

There are many different stretching methods available, but we will use the three most common types – static, dynamic, and tensing and releasing the muscle before stretching, known as contract–relax (CR). All are useful in helping to improve flexibility. The chart on page 26 shows which types of stretching can be used with the exercises in this programme. Further details are shown in Chapter 3.

Static stretching

With static stretching you take your limb to the point where you begin to feel tight, and hold this position. This is the sort of flexibility used in yoga. As the position is held, your tissues are allowed to lengthen gradually, and naturally occurring muscle reflexes help the muscle to relax. This is the most common stretch we will use. All the exercises in phase I and most of those in phases II and III are static stretches.

Static stretching is a particularly safe method. However, because the position may be held for some time, the exercise position must be comfortable and well supported. If you wobble, the stretch may be jerked further, and this is quite dangerous. Lying or sitting on a mat are good positions for static stretches, but kneeling or standing on one leg are not.

Once you have achieved the right position, you need to concentrate on breathing out and 'sighing', because this will allow your muscles to relax further. Hold the stretched position initially for five seconds. Release the stretch and rest for 10–20 seconds to allow blood to flow back into the muscle, and then repeat the stretch. After three sessions of this stretching pattern, increase the holding time to 20–30 seconds, but still perform three repetitions.

After you have been using this stretching pattern for 10–14 days you can extend it to perform five repetitions, holding each for 30 seconds. When the stretch is released after each rep, release the muscle tension slowly, without allowing the tissues to 'spring' back. Recoil of this type can be painful.

The timing stated is for general guidance only. When you stretch, if you feel that holding for 30 seconds is too much, then just release the stretch. We all have off days. One day you might want to stretch more intensely and hold the stretch for longer, while on another day you might want to take it easy. It is more important to listen to your body and respond to its needs than to adhere rigorously to a set time frame.

 KEY POINT
With static stretching make sure you choose a stable body position and try to relax into the movement.

Dynamic stretching

Dynamic stretching simply means stretching while moving. For this type of stretching you end up in more or less the same position as with static stretching, but the idea is to move into this position in a controlled fashion. With dynamic stretching, you are using coordination and what is known as 'muscle sequencing' – that is, one muscle working after another in a specific order. This can be very helpful in sport, where a dynamic stretch can begin to rehearse a sports action, and is especially important when using faster paced running.

To illustrate the difference between static and dynamic stretching, let's take as an example a sprinting action. As you lift your knees high to sprint, your hamstring muscles on the back of your leg are stretched and then contracted as you plant your heel on the ground and 'kick' to get up to speed. You can perform a static stretch for the hamstrings by placing your heel on a table and slowly reaching forwards towards your toes, holding this position as you feel the stretch go on. To perform a dynamic stretch, you could simply use the sprinting action itself, but slow it down so that you take the leg from behind the body and bring it

20

forwards, lifting the knee. This action is similar to that used in the sprint, but you are now performing it in a slow controlled manner.

The key point with dynamic stretching is to maintain control throughout, and to never allow the action to become so rapid that you risk injury. Normally, a total movement in dynamic stretching should take about 10–15 seconds. If the action speeds up so that it only takes two–three seconds, the chances are that it is too fast – you should stop, rest, and begin again at a slower pace.

 KEY POINT
Dynamic stretching is stretching with movement.
It works several muscle groups in sequence.

Contract–relax

Contract–relax (CR) is a form of intense stretching designed to get the maximum stretch by using muscle reflexes. After you tense a muscle – a so-called *isometric* contraction – the muscle relaxes slightly so that its firmness (tone) is less tense than before. We use this fact in CR stretching. First we contract (tense) the muscle, then hold it for two to five seconds, and then relax. During the relaxation period, we stretch.

Nearly all the static stretches that we use in this programme can be converted to CR stretches if you want to take the stretch slightly further. This would be appropriate only after you have practised a stretch for several training sessions, or if you are used to stretching in general and would classify yourself as stretching at an advanced level.

Let's use a common hamstring stretch as an example. Lie on your back on the floor and lift your right leg, keeping it straight. Grasp your leg around your thigh and gently pull your straight leg towards you. Hold this position, breathing normally, and feel the leg muscles on the back of the thigh (hamstrings) gradually release their tension. This is a *static* stretch, because you are simply holding the position.

To add CR stretching to this exercise, keep your hands still, and press your leg downwards (hip extension) against the resistance of your hands. Your leg pushes down and your hands pull up, so nothing actually moves (an isometric contraction), but your hamstring muscles over the back of your thigh tense. Hold this muscle tension for five seconds and then release the tension, allowing your leg to lower slightly. Have a breather for 5–10 seconds, and then perform the static stretch again (pulling your leg up using only your hands, but keeping the leg muscles relaxed). You should now see that you can lift your leg slightly higher, and the feeling in your leg changes. Usually the sharp, slightly painful sensation of the stretch becomes dull and more pleasant. It's a little like taking a kettle off the boil!

Generally, to convert a static stretch into a CR stretch, simply tighten the muscles you are going to stretch, while trying to pull in the opposite direction from the stretch, but without actually allowing movement. To take another example, your calf muscles are stretched by adopting a lunge position where your toes are pulled *upwards* towards your body. To perform CR, you use a toe-pointing action, pulling your toes *downwards* before you stretch.

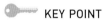 **KEY POINT**
Contract–relax (CR) stretching is intense and can be used to increase the effectiveness of static stretching.
To perform CR, first tense the muscle in the opposite direction from the stretching action.

What to expect from stretching

If you use intensive stretching, either by stretching quite far into your range, or by holding the stretch for longer than about 5–10 seconds, you may find that you are quite sore the next day. Even if you use a fairly brief programme, if it is very intensive you may be as sore as if you had gone for a long run.

There are two reasons for this. Soreness immediately after exercise is due to the build-up of naturally occurring acids within the working muscles. Soreness a day or two after exercise is called *delayed onset muscle soreness*, or DOMS for short. This occurs quite naturally during very intense exercise through minor swelling around the fibres within the stretched muscle. It is quite harmless, but you should not stretch while your muscles are still sore in this way. Instead, use a warm bath and gentle massage to reduce the soreness.

Muscle soreness can also be reduced by using a cool-down after your workout. This should include similar exercises to those you used in your warm-up. The idea is to flush fresh blood through the muscles which have been worked to get rid of the acids which have been building up as you exercise.

Intense stretching is not recommended before running, as it is likely to result in reduced output from the muscles. CR stretching should be an entirely separate part of your training programme.

 KEY POINT

Use a cool-down after exercise to reduce muscle soreness.

Some forms of exercise can give you quite rapid progress. For example, if you weight-train, you can often feel your muscles begin to tone relatively quickly – even within a few weeks. With stretching, however, progress is somewhat slower. It can take two to three months to begin to notice a change, although sometimes progress may be faster. One of the things we aim to do with stretching is to enable a tight muscle to relax. For example, you might have tight, sore shoulder muscles from sitting at a desk all day. When you stretch, you will notice the soreness go quite quickly, but the muscle will not actually lengthen for some months.

Even though progress in stretching can be slow, you will

notice that it is fairly continuous. If you join a yoga class, for example, you will notice that you still continue to improve for some years after you begin. There are obviously physical limitations to progress – if you are 60, no amount of stretching will make you 16 again. However, many people in their sixties find themselves a lot more flexible than they were in their thirties and forties, simply because at the time – often when their children were growing up, and they led busy lives – they did not allow themselves time to exercise and so got into poor physical condition. Now they have time to train and they see progress.

3

Exercises

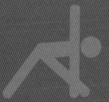

	Exercise	Static	Dynamic	Can CR be added?
	Phase I			
I.1	Hamstrings – active knee extension	✔	✘ ✔	✔
I.2	Rectus femoris stretch – standing	✔	✘	✔
I.3	Calf lunge	✔	✘	✔
I.4	Thoracic spine – sitting	✔	✔	✔
I.5	Spinal rotation – two legs	✔	✔	✔
I.6	Soles of the feet	✔	✘	✘
	Phase II			
II.1	Spinal rotation – lying	✔	✘	✔
II.2	Lower back extension – lying	✔	✔	✘
II.3	Lower back flexion – lying	✔	✔	✘
II.4	Anterior tibials	✔	✘	✘
II.5	Hip adductors – long sitting	✔	✘	✘
II.6	Knee extension – with towel	✔	✘	✔
II.7	Hip flexors – Thomas test	✔	✘	✔
II.8	Iliotibial band	✔	✘	✘
II.9	Deep calf and Achilles	✔	✘	✘
	Phase III			
III.1	Hip adductors – wall support	✔	✘ ✔	✔
III.2	Lateral flexion – standing	✔	✘	✔
III.3	Anterior chest and shoulders	✔	✘	✔
III.4	Gluteals	✔	✘	✘
III.5	Hip flexors – supine lying	✔	✘	✔
III.6	Hamstrings – lying on back	✔	✘	✔
III.7	Leg swing – forwards and backwards	✘	✔	✘
III.8	Leg swing – sideways	✘	✔	✘
III.9	Calf stretch – sprint start	✔	✘ ✔	✘

3. Exercises

Phase I: Beginner

Phase I is the beginning phase. This does not mean you are a beginner to running, but simply that you are stretching in this way for the first time.

We are targeting the muscles used when running, but also using one exercise to loosen the spine. This is important because runners often suffer from stiff, painful backs due to the combination of running posture and jarring, particularly in road running.

This phase lays the foundation for the next two phases, using slightly simpler exercises that are nevertheless very effective. As all the stretches in phase I are static, begin by holding each movement for three to five seconds. Make sure you don't hold your breath, but instead focus your attention on breathing out, as you will often notice that your muscles relax during this time. You can expect your muscles to feel comfortably sore as you stretch, but not painful. If you are very inflexible and the exercises are painful, keep the holding time the same, but release the stretch slightly so that you are pushing just to the beginning of the feeling of stiffness but not right into it. Perform a maximum of two repetitions for each movement.

Generally you can perform all the phase I exercises in a single daily session, but if you are short of time you can perform half in the morning and half in the afternoon. However, remember to do a warm-up before both sessions!

If you were to measure your discomfort on a scale of 1 to 10, with 1 being no discomfort and 10 being very painful indeed, your stretching at the beginning of phase I should only measure 2–3 on the comfort scale.

During the second week you can stretch further into your stiffness range, but even so your discomfort should never be greater than 5 on the scale. Increase the number of reps to three or four, and hold each for 6–10 seconds.

During week three try to hold each rep for 20–30 seconds, and perform five reps. As a guide, a 20–30 second hold corresponds to about five complete breaths (in and out)! This is quite intense stretching now, so it may feel uncomfortable, perhaps 6–7 on the comfort scale. Because you may be sore following this training, perform the exercises on alternate days to allow adequate recovery. You may actually need longer than this to recover. The best guide is not to begin a stretching exercise if the muscles to be stretched are still very sore (above 5 on the comfort scale) from the last session.

Although there are only six exercises in this section, you may find it too time-consuming to perform five reps of each in each training session as recommended for week three. Don't drop any of the exercises, however, as this will leave certain muscles unstretched and risk muscle imbalance. Instead, limit yourself to two well-performed reps.

 KEY POINT

When you are strapped for time, think quality not quantity. Perform two well-executed reps, holding the first for 20 seconds and the second for 30.

SUMMARY – TRAINING IN PHASE I

Week 1
- Hold for 3–5 seconds
- Mild discomfort only
- Two reps per training session
- Daily practice

Week 2
- Hold for 6–10 seconds
- Slight muscle burning
- Three to four reps per training session
- Daily practice

Week 3
- Hold for 20–30 seconds
- Tolerable muscle burning, but NOT PAIN
- Five reps maximum for each exercise
- Alternate days.

Note
Where exercises are described on one side of the body (for example the right leg) you should perform the same exercise on the other side (left leg).

I.1 Hamstrings – active knee extension

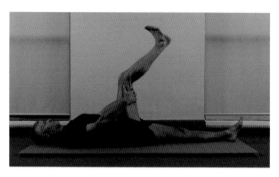

Lie with your back on the floor with your left leg straight and bend your right knee and hip to 90 degrees. Grip your hands behind the right knee and straighten your leg using the power of your quadriceps (the muscle in the front of the thigh) alone. The knee should remain directly above the hip – don't allow it to fall downwards, and your toes should remain relaxed.

Rest for 10 seconds before repeating.

Variations

Place your hand on the front of your leg and actively push the leg on to your hand using the power of your hip muscles; at the same time, extend your knee. This will cause the hamstring muscles (on the back of the leg) to relax further through a natural reflex action. This technique can be useful if your hamstrings are very tight, or if they have a tendency to cramp and go into spasm.

Points to note

- Pulling your toes towards you and flexing your neck will throw stress on to the delicate sciatic nerve running along the back of your leg, and away from the hamstrings. This is a useful procedure in some cases, but is best performed under the supervision of a physiotherapist.

I.2 Rectus femoris stretch – standing

Stand side-on to a wall with your right hand supporting your body weight. Bend your left leg and grip your ankle, keeping your knee bent. Pull your left hip back, while maintaining correct spinal alignment – that is, keeping the natural hollows in the small of your back and the nape of your neck, not rounding or hollowing excessively.

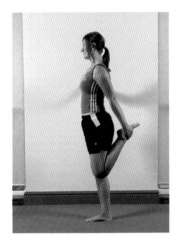

Variations

Loop a towel around your ankle to reduce the amount of knee bend and allow you to pull your hip further back. This will emphasise the upper portion of the muscle.

If this becomes a favourite exercise, you can use it in phases II and III as a CR technique. At the point of maximum stretch, try to straighten your leg at the same time, holding your ankle firmly. Your rectus femoris muscle will tighten and as you release you should find that you can stretch a little further.

Points to note

- The rectus femoris is one of the quadriceps muscles, and acts to extend the leg at the knee. The exercise also stretches the femoral nerve at the front of the thigh.
- A sensation of burning or tingling (pins and needles) over the front of the thigh suggests that this nerve may be tight or possibly trapped, requiring management with physiotherapy.
- Pain in the lower back indicates that you have allowed your back to hollow excessively. Realign your spine and repeat the exercise.

I.3 Calf lunge

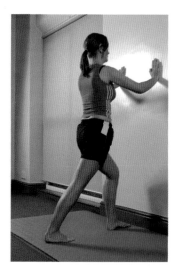

Begin by facing a wall in a half-lunge position with your left foot forward. Place your hands on the wall and bend your arms to lower your body forwards, encouraging your left foot to bend upwards.

Points to note

- Keep your heel on the floor throughout the movement.
- As the knee is straight in this movement, the stretch on the superficial calf muscle (gastrocnemius) is increased and that on the deep calf muscle (soleus) reduced.
- If you are a sprinter your superficial calf muscle may get very tight as it is used powerfully in the sprinting action. This is a vital stretch for you!

Variations

Altering the angle of the foot away from the perpendicular will change the emphasis on the calf muscle. Pressing the knee over the outside of the foot will stretch the inner calf. Pressing it over the inside of the foot stretches the outer calf.

I.4 Thoracic spine – sitting

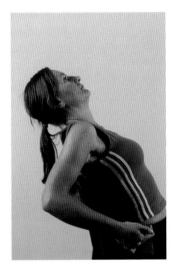

Sit on a high-backed chair with a towel folded over the top of the chair-back for padding. Sit right back in the chair so that your buttocks touch the back. Arch your upper (thoracic) spine over the back of the chair using the padded upper edge as a pivot point. Draw your elbows and upper arms backwards to supply force for the stretch.

Variations

The point on the spine where you feel the stretch will be determined by the contact point between your spine and the edge of the chair-back. Shuffle up and down to place the chair edge higher or lower on the spine until you find the position which gives you the most comfortable stretch.

Points to note

- As you extend your spine backwards, make sure that you do not simply slide your hips forwards, as this will release the stretch and reduce its effectiveness.
- As the spine extends, your ribcage expands, so breathe in at this point.
- Distance runners, this is vital for you! When the mileage builds up and you tire, your shoulders tend to round and your chest slumps. Use this stretch to reverse the body stress this causes.

I.5 Spinal rotation – two legs

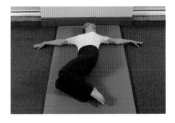

Lie on your back on the floor with your knees and hips bent. Rest your arms on the floor in a T shape. Take your knees to the right side of your body and your head to the left, maintaining the stretch.

The main muscle emphasis of this stretch is on the oblique abdominals which crisscross your trunk, but it also stretches the shoulder and chest muscles. In addition it will release stiffness in the small joints of your lower spine.

Variations

Place a small cushion on the floor and lower your knees onto the cushion to reduce the movement range.

Points to note

- Due to the weight of your legs, they should be lowered slowly; dropping your legs is potentially dangerous to your spine, as it could jolt it.
- It is very common to have asymmetry – where one side of the body is tighter than the other. Hold the stretch to the tighter side for 10 seconds longer to rebalance the body.

- Because distance running causes compression stresses in the lower spine, runners often find their low back very stiff. This exercise is extremely effective at relieving this stiffness and pain, so it will become one of your most important stretches.

I.6 Soles of the feet

With your feet bare, stand in a supported lunge position with your hands against a wall. Gently press the ball of your back foot into a mat, pressing your knee downwards and forwards to encourage your ankle to bend. You are aiming to bend your big toe joint and bring your knee in front of your foot.

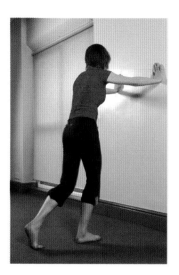

Variations

You can alter the degree of either the knee or toe bend (or both) to vary this stretch.

Points to note

- The plantarfascia is a taut bowstring of tissue which supports the arch of your foot.
- The plantarfascia is tightened by a combination of both toe and ankle bending. Both actions combined are required, and either one performed on its own is less effective.

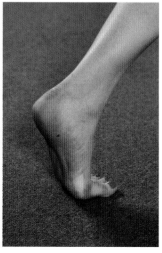

Phase II: Intermediate

In phase II you will stretch a greater variety of muscles, including those used directly in running and areas where tightness builds up in the lower back.

The exercises build on the foundations laid in phase I, and although we are using new exercises, it is fine to swap in any exercises from phase I that you found of particular benefit for your body. It is important that you adapt your training in this way to make your stretching programme more specific to your individual needs.

Begin as before by holding each movement for three to five seconds, focusing on breathing out to help your muscles to relax. You only need to perform a maximum of two repetitions for each movement. As with phase I, pay attention to your discomfort levels. In phase I you did not exceed a score of 2–3 on your comfort scale (10 being the worst possible pain), and in phase II you should aim to score the same or slightly higher, perhaps up to 4, but no more. The term 'no pain, no gain' has little place in modern training programmes. Discomfort is to be expected with intense training, but real pain normally means you have pushed yourself too far and are likely to be injured.

For the second week, stretch further into your stiffness range once more, and increase the number of reps to three or four, with a hold of 6–10 seconds. Finally, in week three, try to hold each rep for 20–30 seconds, performing five reps. As with phase I, in weeks one and two you can perform the exercises daily. In week 3 you may again be quite sore, so stretch on alternate days.

There is no need to perform all the exercises in each session. There are nine exercises in this phase, so try to pick three or four per day so that you have used all nine every two or three days. Splitting the programme up in this way (a method known as periodisation) allows your muscles time to recover. You should aim never to use intense stretching on a muscle which is still sore from a previous training bout. Be guided by what your body tells you as you increase the intensity of your stretching, rather than sticking rigidly to a programme.

SUMMARY – TRAINING IN PHASE II

Week 1
- Hold for 3–5 seconds
- Moderate discomfort only
- Two reps
- Daily training
- Continue to use any phase I exercises you found especially beneficial

Week 2
- Hold for 6–10 seconds
- Slight muscle burning
- Three to four reps
- Daily training

Week 3
- Hold for 20–30 seconds
- Slight muscle burning
- Five reps
- Alternate days.

 KEY POINT

Don't use intense stretching on a muscle which is still sore from a previous training session.

II.1 Spinal rotation – lying

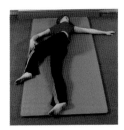

Lie on your back on the floor with your right arm out at 90 degrees. Bend your left knee and twist your trunk towards the right leg, bringing your left knee towards the floor. You will feel the stretch both on your back and on the outside of your hip.

You can put some overpressure on the stretch by pressing your knee to the floor using your right arm. This is a direct progression from exercise I.5. Now, because your bottom leg is straight, you can lower the top leg further towards the ground, increasing the stretch.

Variations

If you find the stretch difficult, place a cushion on the floor and take your knee down onto the cushion; or adjust the degree of bend at your hip and knee to alter the stress of the stretch.

If you get spasms in your back muscles during the day, try converting this into a CR stretch. As you press down on your left knee, twist your trunk and press your right leg upwards against your hand. Press your hand and knee with equal and opposite force so nothing actually moves. Hold for five seconds and then release, allowing the knee to lower to the ground.

One side of the spine is often tighter than the other, especially in track runners who lean into the bend as they run. If this applies to you, perform the stretch to the tighter side for 10 seconds longer than for the unaffected side.

Points to note

- Because this action involves leverage, it should be performed in a slow and controlled manner.
- Your lower hip will tuck under your body as you rotate. This is fine, as it becomes the pivot point around which your body moves.

II.2 Lower back extension – lying

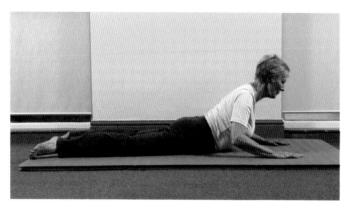

Lie on the floor on your front and place your hands on the floor in the press-up position. Slowly push with your arms to arch your spine, keeping your hips firmly on the floor. Pause in the upper position and then lower.

This movement stretches the rectus abdominis muscle on the front of your tummy. It also corrects any pressure in the spongy discs in your lower back, which is often brought on by prolonged sitting or lifting.

Variations

Pushing from your forearms until your elbows are locked at 90 degrees will limit the movement range; pulling your arms towards your shoulders will increase this range. Choose an arm position which is comfortable for you.

Points to note

- This movement should be encouraged rather than forced, and repeated rhythmically to gain a pumping action on the discs of your lower spine.
- You should feel the stretch, but not pain, in the lower back. If you experience pain, stop immediately.

II.3 Lower back flexion – lying

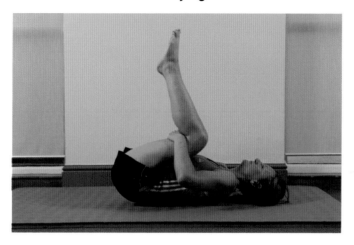

Lie on your back on the floor, drawing your knees up to your chest. Grip your knees and pull them into your chest and up towards your shoulders. This position should create a rocking position in your lower back, which will stretch your lower back muscles (the erector spinae).

Variations

Combine this movement with twisting (rotation) or side bending to subtly alter the stress on your spine.

Points to note

• The movement is one of pulling your knees towards your shoulders rather than pulling them in towards your chest.

II.4 Anterior tibials

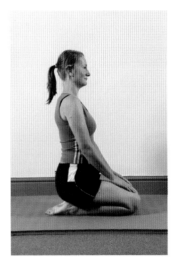

Kneel on the floor and then sit back on your ankles, pressing the front of the ankles to the floor.

You should feel a stretch along the outside of your shin bone (the anterior tibial muscles).

Variations

Place a folded towel beneath your toes to press them into flexion and increase the stretch on the toe extensor muscles.

Points to note

- This exercise can place considerable stress on your knees. If you have knee pain, perform the exercise leaning on a stool to support your body weight.
- If you have ever suffered from a broken ankle, you may not be able to perform this exercise. You will feel the stretch on your stiff ankle rather than on your shin muscles. See a physiotherapist to determine which ankle stretching exercises are appropriate for your condition.

II.5 Hip adductors – long sitting

Sit on the floor with both legs straight. You should have your back flat against a wall, with a rolled towel placed in the small of your back (lumbar area) to maintain spinal alignment. Bend your right leg, placing the foot on your left thigh above the knee. Support your foot with your left hand, and press down on your right knee with your right hand.

You should feel this stretch on the inside of your thigh, travelling up into the groin. Lengthen your spine and maintain good spinal alignment throughout the movement.

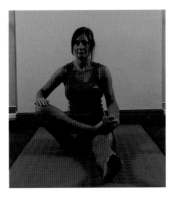

Points to note

- Most individuals will find that one leg is more flexible than the other.
- Those with reduced flexibility of the muscles on the inside of the thigh may tend to tilt the body towards the bent knee, lifting the pelvis and buttock from the floor. This gives an apparent increase in flexibility as the knee can be lowered further, but in fact does not create any more stretch in these muscles.
- Do not perform this exercise (except under the supervision of a physiotherapist) if you have suffered from Pubic Symphasis Dysfunction (PSD) after recent childbirth.

Variations

You can also sit on a wedge to tip your pelvis forwards. If your knee is too stiff to bend enough to allow your foot to rest on your thigh, rest your foot on the shin just below your knee instead.

41

II.6 Knee extension – with towel

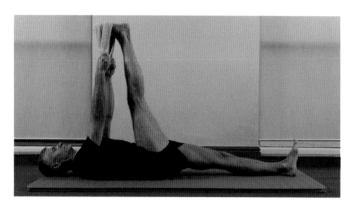

Lie with your back on the floor with your left leg straight, and bend your right knee and hip to an angle of 90 degrees from the floor. Hook a folded towel around your right foot, holding one end of the towel in each hand. Now try to straighten your leg by pushing your foot into the towel. Do not allow your arms to straighten, and keep the hip, knee and foot in a straight line.

Variations

Instead of a towel, use an exercise band. Make sure the band is in the centre of the foot rather than around the toes to prevent it from slipping.

Points to note

- Fastening the towel over your toes will pull the toes towards you.
- Combining this movement with bending (flexion) of the neck will throw stress on to the nerves and away from the hamstring muscles. This is a technique often used by physiotherapists to stretch a tight nerve after injury. Although useful, you should not continue the stretch if you get pins and needles in your leg, as this means too much stress is being placed on the nerve.

II.7 Hip flexors – Thomas test position

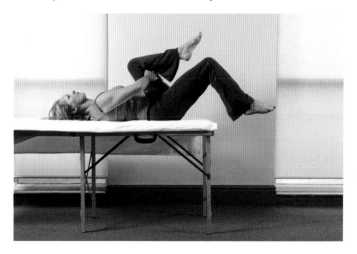

Lie with your back on a bench or stable dining table and your right leg over the bench end. Bend your left hip and knee and pull your knee towards your chest. You will feel the stretch on the lower leg, along the front of the thigh and up into the front of the hip.

Variations

Start with both knees bent and the feet flat on the bench. Pull one knee to the chest and then lower the opposite leg.

Points to note

• This movement is known as the Thomas test, a test used in physiotherapy to assess hip flexor muscle tightness.

II.8 Iliotibial band (ITB)

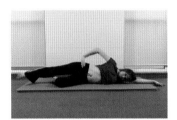

This movement stretches a tight band (the ITB) which runs down the outside of your leg from pelvis to knee (see page 73). The band can get very tight in runners and particularly needs stretching to protect against overuse injury in endurance running.

Lie on your left side with your left leg slightly bent for support. Lift your right leg upwards and sideways. Pressing the left side of your body firmly into the mat, allow the upper leg to lower slowly onto the mat. You should feel a stretch over the outside of the hip and on the upper outer edge of the thigh.

Variations

Allowing your leg to move forwards or backwards alters the effect of this movement. Taking it forwards targets the ITB alongside the smaller buttock (gluteal) muscles; taking it backwards stretches the ITB with the hip muscles.

You can also try the exercise with a partner pressing gently down on the top of your pelvis (not your hip joint) as you stretch the leg. This prevents movement at the pelvis, so throwing all the stretch onto the ITB itself.

Points to note

- The aim is to drop the top hip without letting your pelvis tilt sideways. This is achieved by flattening the side of the trunk against the mat. If your pelvis moves, even slightly, the stretch will be ineffective.
- Only when the ITB is tight do you feel the stretch over the outside of the hip; if your ITB is flexible, you may not notice this.

II.9 Deep calf and Achilles

Place a low stool or chair against a wall to stop it sliding. Put your left foot in the centre of the chair, place your right foot on the floor and slightly to the side of the chair, and take up a lunge position. Keeping your foot flat, and your heel in contact with the chair seat, press your knee forwards over your toes.

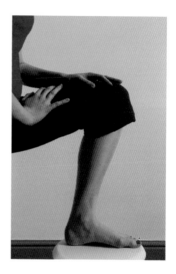

Variations

Altering the angle of the foot away from the perpendicular will change the emphasis on the deep calf and Achilles.

By bending the knee, the emphasis is taken away from the long superficial calf muscle (gastrocnemius) and placed on the shorter, deep calf muscles (soleus and tibialis posterior). This is a useful alternative to try once each week for variety.

Points to note

- Your heel must remain on the chair seat throughout the movement. Raising the heel takes the emphasis away from the deep calf and Achilles and throws it onto the foot itself.

Phase III: Advanced

Phase III maintains the theme of the previous phases: the exercises here target both the muscles involved in running, and those body areas which tend to get stiff due to the running posture. As well as the spine, you will also be stretching out the chest and shoulders as this area tends to tighten if runners develop a round-shouldered posture. This can often give a burning pain between the shoulder blades, so it is an important factor to address.

In addition to the static stretches seen in phases I and II, we are now introducing dynamic stretches in preparation for more explosive actions such as sprinting and 'kicking' at the end of a race or intense training run.

In this phase we perform the programme with the same repetitions and holding times as phases I and II. However, the phase III movements are generally more challenging, so make sure you really focus on good exercise technique. Make sure you don't bounce into the movements or hold your breath. Be sure to follow the exercise instructions closely and be aware of your body alignment. In phases I and II we took three weeks to complete the whole phase. For phase III, you may use this weekly timing as a guide, but because the exercises are more advanced, it is best to progress only when you are ready.

Begin holding each movement for three to five seconds, and perform two reps of each movement. Progress to three or four reps, with a hold for 6–10 seconds, when you feel ready. Select the exercises which you find most beneficial and perform these, holding each rep for 20–30 seconds and performing five reps.

How will you know when you are ready to move on? Remember first that you must not stretch if you are still sore from the day before. If you are not sore, try to hold the movement for longer (except if you are performing a stretch dynamically of course). If you can hold the stretch correctly without wobbling or feeling that it is very painful (8 on the comfort scale) you are ready to move on.

There are again nine exercises in phase III, so pick three or four per day so that you use all nine every two to three days.

You may now consider increasing the intensity of your stretching by adding some contract–relax (CR) movements after you have performed two reps of your static stretching. The exercise descriptions explain how to do this.

SUMMARY – TRAINING IN PHASE III

To begin:
- Hold for 3–5 seconds
- Moderate discomfort only
- Two reps

Progress when ready to:
- Holding for 6–10 seconds
- Slight muscle burning
- Three to four reps

Progress when ready to:
- Holding for 20–30 seconds
- Slight muscle burning
- Five reps
- Consider using CR stretching where appropriate.

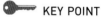 **KEY POINT**

Phase III training is more intense, but make sure you keep each movement under control.

III.1 Hip adductors – wall support

Lie with your back on the floor with your legs straight up in the air and your buttocks close to a wall. Rest your legs against the wall and allow them to lower slowly out to the sides and downwards (this is known as hip abduction). You should feel the stretch on the inside of the thigh right up into the groin. Hold this position (static stretch) for 20–30 seconds and then bring your legs back up again by 20–30 cm (resisted adduction), before again allowing them to lower.

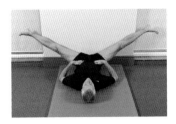

Variations

Lifting the legs against their own weight provides resistance for contract–relax (CR) stretching. This resistance can be increased by having a training partner resist the adduction movement for you by pressing down on your legs.

If you perform this action rhythmically – one rep per complete movement – the action becomes a dynamic stretch. In this case, you do not hold the fully stretched position (legs in the lower position) but instead lift the legs up again straight away. This is a useful variation to put in perhaps once each week.

Points to note

- Although this is obviously a stretching exercise, because the legs are lifted against their own weight you will also gain adductor muscle strength.

III.2 Lateral flexion – standing

Stand with your feet shoulder width apart. Bend your spine sideways (side flexion), placing your right arm on your waist or thigh to support your body weight. Take your left arm above your head to increase the stretch.

This movement stretches the side bending muscles on the upper (left) side of the body.

Right   Wrong

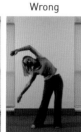

Variations

Place both arms on your waist to reduce the load. Stretching both hands overhead increases the overload on the spine, and changes the emphasis of the exercise from stretch to strength.

Points to note

- Asymmetry of the side bending action of the spine is common, so you may find that your degree of movement is greater on one side than the other.
- The photograph on the left shows the exercise being performed correctly: the subject's right hand is on her hip, taking the weight of her trunk, and the curve of her spine is gentle. In the right-hand photo the subject has not placed her hand on her waist for support. As her whole upper bodyweight is now pressing down on the spine, she has bent further but the curve of her spine is no longer gentle. In addition, because her body is forced further down her right hip is now pressed sideways and she no longer takes her weight equally over both feet – her posture is less stable and she could easily topple over.

III.3 Anterior chest and shoulders

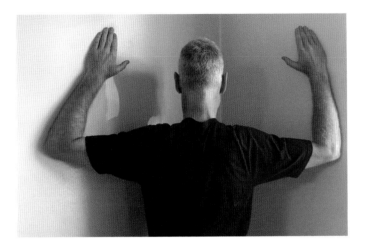

Stand facing a doorway or corner of a room with your upper arms out to your sides at shoulder level and elbows bent at 90 degrees. Lean forwards, pressing your chest through the doorway or into the corner, and forcing your arms back into extension. You should feel the stretch over the front of your chest.

Variations

Increasing and reducing the height of your arms will vary the focus of the stretch.

Points to note

- Because the full body weight is being supported by your upper body, heavy individuals and those with poor shoulder flexibility should take up a lunge position, moving some of the body weight on to the front foot.

III.4 Gluteals

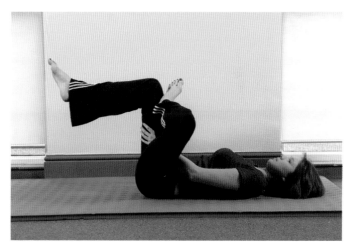

Lie with your back on the floor. Bend your left leg at the hip and knee – about a 90 degree angle at each. Then draw your right knee up, pressing it on to your left foot. Reach around your right knee or thigh and pull your knee towards your right shoulder, pressing your left hip into an outward twisting position (external rotation). You should feel a stretch in your buttock and on the outside of your left hip.

Variations

Altering the position of your left leg (either by twisting it more or less, or pulling it up more or less) will change the emphasis of the stretch. Alter the leg position so that you feel comfortable when holding the stretch.

Points to note

- This exercise also places stress on the pelvis, so it should not be used for three months after childbirth.
- If you are unable to bend your hip high enough to grip around your thigh, loop a towel around your thigh and grip that instead.

III.5 Hip flexors – supine lying (with partner)

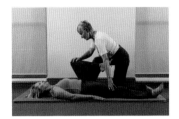

Lie on the floor on your back, with your left hip and knee bent. Your partner should half kneel at your left hip. With her left hand she holds your right leg on the floor, and with her right hand presses your left leg closer to your chest (hip flexion).

This movement stretches the hip flexor muscles of the lower leg, and the buttock of the upper leg.

Variations

If you experience pain in your flexed knee, your partner should place her hand on the underside of the knee, to avoid compressing the joint.

If you do not have a partner, you can perform the exercise yourself, simply pulling your own knee to your chest. The advantage of having a partner do this for you, however, is that you are able to relax all your muscles as the stretch is put on.

Points to note

- Most individuals are asymmetrical, so one leg may appear less flexible than the other.
- Do not perform this stretch if you have had a hip joint replacement.

III.6 Hamstrings – lying on back (with partner)

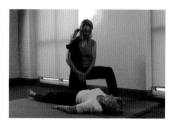

Lie on the floor on your back, with your legs straight. Your partner should half kneel at your right hip and lift your right leg, placing her hand over your right knee to keep the leg straight. With your leg resting on your partner's shoulder she should lunge forwards, pressing your leg further upwards (hip flexion). Hold this stretched position (static stretch) by trying to relax your leg on your partner's shoulder. Slowly release the stretch as your partner lowers your leg.

Variations

Place a small pad on your partner's shoulder and a small rolled towel under your back to make the position more comfortable.

To increase the stretch further, use a CR technique. With your partner holding your leg, press the leg downwards (hip extension) as your partner presses against you. Tense the muscles without any movement (isometric contraction) and as you relax, have your partner press your leg further upwards, performing the static stretch described above.

Points to note

• When locking your leg out straight, make sure that the pressure is not placed directly over your kneecap. Your partner should cup her hand and place it around, but not directly on top of, your knee.

III.7 Leg swing – forwards and backwards

Stand with your feet shoulder width apart. Hold on to a bar or the frame of a piece of gym apparatus or furniture at your right side for balance. Swing your left leg forwards and upwards (hip flexion), first to shin level, then to waist level and eventually to chest level. You will feel the stretch on the back of your thigh (hamstring muscles) as your leg swings forwards, and on the front of the thigh (hip flexors) as it swings backwards.

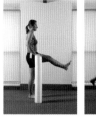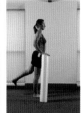

Progress the range of motion as you feel comfortable, being careful not to overstretch. As your leg goes backwards, maintain your lower back alignment – do not allow your back to hollow excessively.

Variations

Keeping the leg straight places the stretch on the hip. If you let the knee bend, as though kicking your backside, you will stretch the thigh muscles right down to your knee as well.

Points to note

- Make sure the action is controlled throughout the movement range.
- Do not allow the momentum to pull you into a range that you would not normally use.
- Too much speed will force your pelvis to tip forwards, hollowing your back excessively.

III.8 Leg swing – sideways

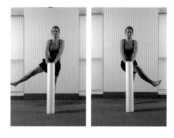

Stand facing a piece of gym equipment or high cupboard with your feet hip width apart. Hold on with both hands, shift your pelvis to the left to take your weight onto your left leg, and unload your right. Swing your right leg out to the side and then inwards and in front of the left leg. Start by swinging outwards to shin level, then knee and finally hip level. As you swing, do not allow your trunk to twist.

As the leg swings outwards, you will feel the stretch on the inside of your thigh up to your groin and as it swings inwards you will feel it over the outside of the hip and thigh.

Variations

Pointing your heel to the ceiling (toes to the floor) combines swinging outwards with twisting inwards. Pointing your toes to the ceiling combines hip rotation with a sideways twist. Twisting actions – which work the hip rotator muscles that lie beneath your powerful gluteals (buttocks) – are important because they also help to stabilise the joint. Use both leg actions to balance your training programme unless you already have a good inward twist, in which case focus on the lateral rotation movement. With this variation, you may also feel the stretch deep inside the hip joint.

Points to note

- To unload the swinging leg, you must transfer your body weight over the other (weight-bearing) leg. You can achieve this by shifting your pelvis over the weight-bearing leg.
- If you lack hip control and hip stability, you may find that you simply tip your spine sideways. Try to avoid this by keeping your spine upright and your pelvis level.

III.9 Calf stretch – sprint start

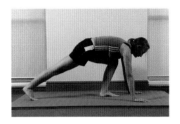

Stand in a lunge position with your right leg back and your left leg forwards, with your weight over your front leg. Place the toes of your back foot on the ground and gradually take your weight backwards, forcing your heel onto the ground as you do so. Pause, then use the calf strength of your back leg to 'flick' you forwards as though exploding out of the blocks from a sprint start. Repeat the exercise five times with the right leg back, then reverse the movement.

Variations

Placing your back leg further back will increase the intensity of the stretch; taking your leg further forwards will reduce it.

You can emphasise the power aspect of this movement rather than the stretch by taking more weight on to your back leg and jumping slightly as you flick yourself forwards. This then becomes a dynamic stretch. Use this if you have suffered from a calf injury after you have had physiotherapy treatment and used static stretching for four to six weeks. Before you run again, the dynamic stretch will prepare you for explosive actions such as suddenly lengthening your pace, or exploding out of the blocks on a track.

Points to note

• Make sure you build the range of motion progressively. Start with your feet quite close together and gradually move your back leg further backwards as your confidence in the movement grows.

56

Maintaining your flexibility

When you have completed all three phases of the programme, you will have built up to intense stretching over about a nine- or ten-week period. You now have a choice – to maintain your current stretching level, or to continue to develop further flexibility on problem areas. If you found any of the exercises really hard, and were not able to stretch to the degree you would like, continue with these movements. Practise these at the beginning of your stretching workout when you are fresh.

   To maintain your new-found level of flexibility, pick three exercises from the programme and practise these daily, changing the three you select each day. Rest from stretching for either one day per week or two if you find you are very sore. In this way you will be using a total of 15 or 18 different stretching exercises each week and maintaining your level of flexibility with a good variety of movements.

   If you find this too demanding, you should stretch a minimum of three times per week using the following exercises:

   • Exercise I.1: hamstrings – active knee extension
   • Exercise I.2: rectus femoris stretch – standing
   • Exercise I.3: calf lunge
   • Exercise II.5: hip adductors – long sitting.

Use alternate days (Monday, Wednesday and Friday, for example) and practise each of the exercises in a single session. As part of your preparation for a run, you can use these stretches following a general warm-up. If you are simply going for a light jog, use the stretches before you go out, and then walk to loosen off before your run. In this case, use static stretching, holding each stretch for three to five seconds only, and perform each movement twice. If you are stretching on a day when you will not run, you can increase the holding time to 20–30 seconds and perform four or five reps of each exercise, after performing a warm-up intense enough to cause you to sweat lightly.

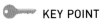
During this three day period, swelling is still forming. After
this, probably no fresh swelling will develop, so although your
ankle stills appears swollen, it is old swelling rather than new.
Once the swelling has stopped forming, you can stop using the
ice.

Compression
Swelling is caused by a sticky fluid, which if unchecked will
spread over the tissues near the injury and stick them together,
making the area stiff. To prevent this, use compression. The
simplest method is an elastic tubular bandage from a chemist. If
you don't have one, wrap a standard crepe bandage around the
ankle. Failing this, use a tea towel instead. The compression
should be comfortable: if you feel your ankle throbbing, it is
probably too tight, so remove it and re-apply it slightly less tightly.

Elevation
With lower limb injuries (those to the ankle, knee or hip) the
watery swelling tends to be pulled down by gravity and form a
thick pool around your ankle bones. To prevent this, rest with
your leg up or elevated on a stool. Raise it at least to the
horizontal or slightly above. This will make your return to
running far quicker.
Elevate your leg for three days after injury, while swelling is
forming. Later, if you find your leg has a tendency to swell if
you do too much on it, you can still use elevation to reduce the
swelling at any time. If the swelling is stubborn a good trick is
to put a cushion between your mattress and bed base at night.
This will provide a few inches of elevation, which is not enough
to stop you sleeping, but just enough to reduce the swelling
overnight.

Getting back into running

Once the pain and swelling begin to ease (about three to five days after injury) you can begin very gentle exercise to help loosen the stiff tissues. The trick is to get a balance between doing just enough to ease the stiffness, but not too much so that you disrupt the healing tissues. The guide here is pain. If you begin with pain and it gradually eases, the chances are that you are simply easing off some stiffness. However, if the pain begins to increase, you should stop, as it means you are doing too much and the tissues will start to swell again. The golden rule of rehabilitation (exercise following injury) is never to exercise through increasing pain.

 KEY POINT

Never exercise through increasing pain.

Begin with simple, non-weight-bearing movements, that is, without taking your weight through the injury. In the case of the ankle, for example, gently circle the ankle and flex it up and down. For a knee, sit on a table or stool and slowly bend and straighten your knee. As you feel the movement tightening, gradually try to ease into the stiff region. If the movement slowly begins to increase, that's fine – you can continue for 5–10 reps and then rest. Have a breather and then start again, aiming to perform two sets of 10 reps twice each day.

About one or two weeks after the injury you will be ready to use stretching exercises. Remember the golden rule not to work through increasing pain. Remember also that stretching, although the topic of this book, is not the only fitness component you should work on during a rehabilitation programme. You will need to re-strengthen your injured limb and also build up the muscle endurance. An important factor following any injury is stability of the limb – how capable your muscles are of supporting your joint and holding it firm. This, combined with exercises to develop the sense of balance in the limb, is often the final deciding factor between getting back into running and suffering setbacks.

It is always best to perform your rehabilitation under the guidance of a qualified physiotherapist. An expert will often see things about your injury that you cannot, so a visit to your physio is a good investment.

Let's have a look now at some specific running injuries and the best stretching exercises to use to aid recovery.

Sprained ankle

When you sprain your ankle, you are most likely to injure the ligament on the outside of the joint. This structure supports your ankle when it points in and down, and following injury it is often this movement which is tight and so needs to be stretched again.

The easiest way to stretch this area is to cross your injured leg at the shin over the uninjured one, then use one hand to steady the lower leg on the injured side, and cup the other around the foot and ankle to pull it down, round and inwards. The stretch should be gentle and held for 5–10 seconds, providing this does not increase the pain.

Once you have managed this, the next stage is to stretch your ankle actively by standing and rocking over on to the outer edge of your foot, or by walking on a slope. This movement is still slow and controlled, but eventually you can use faster actions to develop agility (stretch, balance and strength combined) in the ankle structures. One of the best ways to achieve an agile ankle joint is to walk on an uneven surface such as soft ground or sand. You can also make your own uneven surface by placing four or five cushions on the ground and walking, then slowly jogging, over them in bare feet. At each stage, the action must be controlled, so you don't feel that the movement is 'running away' with you.

As well as stretching the side of the ankle, walking on an

uneven surface also strengthens the muscles surrounding the ankle so that they can support or stabilise the joint. Ankle stability is the most important aspect of fitness to develop following an ankle injury.

Another way to work on stability of this type is to stand on one leg (the injured one) and hold this position for 20–30 seconds. When you do this, you will notice all the muscles around the ankle 'flickering' as they work hard to support the joint and hold it stable.

 KEY POINT

Following a sprained ankle, stretch the outside of the joint and stabilise it using single-leg standing actions.

Shin splints

Shin splints is a condition affecting the shin muscles themselves. These are long muscles running alongside the two shin bones (the tibia and fibula). The muscles are sandwiched between the tight skin of your shin and the flat shin bones. With training, the muscles swell and thicken and, as this happens, they are unable to expand fully because of their sandwiched position. Instead of expanding, pressure within them increases, which cuts off their own blood supply. This reduction in blood flow, combined with a build-up of acids within the muscles, gives rise to the characteristic gnawing pain of shin splints.

Stretching exercises can help some types of shin splints by preventing the muscles from becoming short and tight in the first place.

On the front of the shin lie two sets of muscles, the anterior tibials and the toe extensors. These muscles pull the foot and toes upwards, an action used repeatedly as you run. To stretch

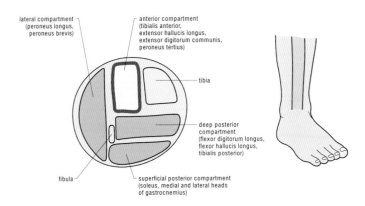

Compartments of the lower leg

these muscles, immediately after running, you should press the foot slowly downwards in the opposite direction, using exercise II.4. To increase the stretch on your toes, place a folded towel on the floor beneath them, which will cause your toes to bend further and so stretch your shin muscles more. Hold this stretch for 30–60 seconds to allow the muscles to 'give' gradually.

Repeat the stretch four or five times after each run.

Pulled hamstring

Areas of injury in a muscle

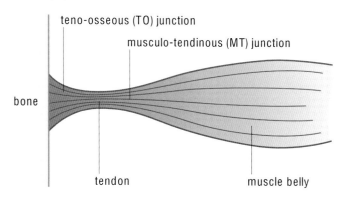

teno-osseous (TO) junction

musculo-tendinous (MT) junction

bone

tendon

muscle belly

When you tear a hamstring, you may injure the muscle in its centre part (called the belly) or at the end of the muscle (called the muscle-tendon or MT junction). The difference between these two areas is that the MT junction does not contract, while the muscle belly does. As well as stretching, muscle-belly tears will therefore need strength training to broaden the muscle and separate the individual muscle fibres to prevent them from sticking together. Injury to the MT junction often responds to stretching alone.

Because the hamstring muscles are involved in all types of running actions, you will need to use two types of stretches – static to regain the movement range, and dynamic to build up the 'whipping' action of the muscle.

Use exercise I.1 to begin. Once this is comfortable, progress to the long sitting exercise shown opposite. You may use both exercises to begin with, but when you stretch for a longer period (20–30 second hold) use only the long sitting exercise.

Hamstring stretch – long sitting exercise

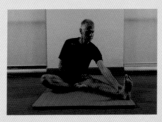 Sit with your injured leg straight and your other leg comfortably bent. Reach forwards with your hand on the side of the straight leg to grip your shin or foot. Press the other hand on your straightened knee to maintain knee extension. Make sure you maintain spinal alignment by gently curving through the spine.

Ease into the movement, gradually increasing your movement range. Hold the comfortably stretched position initially for 10–15 seconds and then for 20–30 seconds; perform four or five reps. You should also perform some of the stretches with the knee slightly unlocked (bent). This will take the stretch away from the lower hamstrings and you will feel the stretch more focused on the upper muscle portion towards your buttock.

To redevelop the hamstring's 'whipping' action, use the dynamic leg swinging exercise (III.7). Swing your leg initially to shin level and then to waist and finally chest height. Begin slowly and gradually build up speed. Once you are confident with this single direction movement (up and down), change to a multi-direction movement, kicking across the body (up, down and across) and then build in twisting actions.

The final stage of rehabilitation is to use more intense running-based exercise:

- Begin with a slow jog, building speed and striding out.
- Rest, and then move on to mid-pace striding from rest.
- Progress to small sprints initially from a running pace and then from rest.
- Use actions such as sprint starts and finally zigzag and backwards running, which will work the hamstrings in slightly different ways.

 KEY POINT

The hamstrings perform fast whipping actions as you run. Begin with slow static stretching and build to dynamic stretching exercises and running drills.

Swollen knee

When the knee suffers a minor injury, it swells and limits the movement of the joint. As the swelling clots and the injury heals, movements will feel stiff and the knee may give way if it is unable to straighten completely. For this reason you need to work both the bending (flexion) and straightening (extension) movements of the knee. From these relatively simple movements you can finally progress to agility-based actions involving twisting, which also help to build confidence in the knee. This latter feature is often overlooked, but it is very important, especially if the knee has been giving way.

Begin your rehab programme using the rectus femoris stretch (I.2), but instead of pulling the thigh backwards level with the hip, allow the thigh to move forwards to take the stretch away from the muscles and redirect it to the joint. To work on straightening, use exercise II.6, stretching the hamstrings with a towel. Again, refocus the exercise by allowing the thigh to move downwards, so as to release the hamstring stretch and focus instead on locking the knee out fully. Once you are confident with these actions, move on.

Developing agility in the knee: (a) grapevine movement to place sideways strain on the knee; (b) increasing range of movement

For the next movement, try the following:
- Stand with your feet shoulder width apart.
- Step forwards and across with the uninjured leg so that the stress is taken on the injured knee.
- Step backwards and across to place the opposite stress on the joint – see (a) in the diagram.

This action can be used as a side-step to perform a 'grapevine' action, stepping first in front of and then behind the injured leg. Bending the knee further will increase the stress on the knee, and performing the action over a bench to bend the knee to near maximum will test the knee fully – see (b) in the diagram. Be cautious, however, because these actions stress the knee considerably, so must be carefully controlled. You are now working for stretch, strength and balance of the knee all at the same time (agility).

Groin strain

Groin strain is a common injury in sprinting, and in cross country if you suddenly slip, pulling your foot sideways. There are two types of groin muscles, or adductors – the long adductors travel from the groin right down to the knee, and the short adductors go from the groin to the upper thigh only. Two exercises are useful for this area, one for the short adductor muscles and the other for the long.

Hip adductor stretches for groin strain

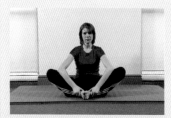

- Begin by sitting on the floor with the soles of your feet together.
- Holding your feet with both hands, press down on your knees or thighs to push them apart.

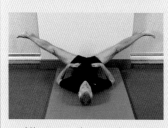

The second stretch (similar to exercise III.1) emphasises the long adductor:
- Lie on your back with your legs straight against a wall.
- Part your legs as far as possible.
- Allow your legs to lower slowly and hold this position.

In both exercises, contract–relax (CR) stretching may be used (see page 21). For this, apply resistance while lifting your legs (press down on your knees in the first stretch, and lift against gravity in the second). Hold the tensed position for 5–10 seconds and then lower your legs again to increase the stretch still further.

It is important when you are rehabilitating after groin strain that strength training and stretching go hand in hand. As the stretching feels easier, use dynamic movements. This can be done in a swimming pool with breaststroke-type actions, or in the gym using elastic tubing. In addition, jogging, cutting, side stepping and zigzag running drills constitute dynamic stretching and also prepare the muscle for running sports.

 KEY POINT

Following a groin injury, static stretches should be performed both with the knee bent and with it straight. Later, move on to dynamic stretching, and stepping/running drills.

Clicking hip and clicking knee

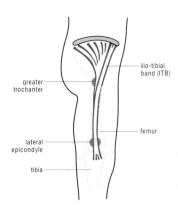

The iliotibial band (ITB)

Clicking hip and clicking knee are two conditions that can result from tightness in the strong band of tissue which runs along the outside of the leg, known as the iliotibial band or ITB.

At its upper end, the ITB attaches to the hip muscles and then passes over a knobble of bone called the greater trochanter at the top of the thighbone (femur). As the leg is moved forwards and backwards, the ITB passes in front of and behind this knobble. If it is tight, the ITB will flick over the knobble like a guitar string. This causes pain and swelling, and often a clicking sensation that can be felt and, in extreme cases, actually heard.

A similar mechanism exists at the knee, where the ITB can flick over a point of bone on the lower end of the thighbone called the lateral epicondyle. The painful clicking sensation that occurs here is often called 'runner's knee'.

ITB stretching will reduce the chance of these conditions occurring, or lessen the pain if they already exist. The exercise shown below is designed to stretch the ITB by holding the pelvis still and pulling the hip inwards. Initially, use only three reps, holding each for five seconds, and perform the movement daily. As your flexibility improves keep to the same number of reps, but build up the holding time to 20–30 seconds.

The upper portion of the ITB at the hip may also be isolated using exercise II.8. Again, the pelvis is held still while the hip is moved inwards. This time, however, the knee is bent, releasing the stretch in the lower portion of the ITB and throwing greater stress on the upper portion.

The upper ITB

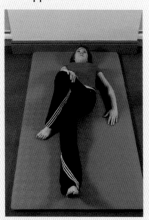

- Lie on your back on a mat.
- Keeping your right foot on the floor, bend your right leg to 90 degrees at the knee and hook your left calf over the top of it.
- Grip the upper rim of your pelvis with your right hand and, holding your pelvis down on the mat, use your left leg to press your right hip inwards.
- Hold for 30–40 seconds, then repeat on the other side.

You should feel the stretch over the outside of the hip and on the upper outer edge of the thigh.

74

The calf and Achilles

When the Achilles tendon is injured, you should perform calf stretches with your knee flexed (see exercise I.3). When the calf is injured, however, it is usually the long calf muscle (gastrocnemius) that is affected, and you should stretch with the knee straight.

When you can perform this statically without pain, use the exercise shown below.

As you return to running, use gentle jogging to begin with and build up the pace gradually. Remember also that running uphill will place a greater stretch on the calf, so be cautious, and when your muscles are tired try not to finish on an uphill run.

Calf and Achilles stretch

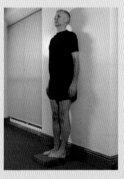

- Stand on a 5 cm block (a thick book or yoga block) and place the ball of your foot on the back edge.
- Allow the heel to lower down, keeping the knee locked – this will stretch the long calf muscle.
- Starting from standing again, raise up on to your toes against your body weight.

Initially, you should hold onto something to take some of your body weight off the calf. Eventually, full body-weight can be used and the exercise can be speeded up until faster, more explosive actions are used to work the muscle intensely.

The arch of the foot

Although running shoes are well padded and have foot-contoured insoles, you may still suffer from arch pain at some stage. Frequently, this affects the cord-like structure which stretches from the heel to the ball of the foot – the plantarfascia. If this structure becomes inflamed or damaged, stretching can help once pain begins to settle.

Use the exercise shown below to bend both the toes and ankle simultaneously. The plantarfascia will stand out as a tight cord in the sole of the foot.

After suffering from pain in the foot, it is wise to check out your training shoes and to visit a physiotherapist or podiatrist to see if you need a special orthotic insole made which is contoured to your particular foot type.

Toe and ankle bend

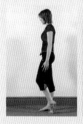 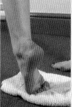

- With your feet bare, stand with one hand against a wall.
- Point the foot furthest from the wall and press the ball of the foot into a mat (left), forcing your toes to bend upwards.
- Hold for 20–30 seconds then release.
- Pause, then press the backs of your toes into the mat (right), encouraging your toes to bend downwards.
- Perform three reps.

If you find this stretch uncomfortable, press your toes onto a cushion or folded towel placed on the mat.

Getting the balance right

Remember that the use of stretching for sports injuries should be *progressive*. This means that as you heal, you can stretch that little bit further or move a little faster. However, always bear in mind that this is a balance. You must do enough to help your body heal correctly, but not too much, in case you tear the healing tissues. Let pain be your guide here. If a stretch causes slight aching, that is fine, but if you feel pain, stop, rest and re-start the next day.

Remember also that running is a skill, and the skill is your running style or gait. After any injury make sure that you run evenly. Have your training partner look at you running from in front, the side and behind.

• Are your steps even or is one longer than the other?
• Do you throw one foot out compared to the other?
• Does your knee move over your foot or does one leg (or both) appear knock-kneed or bow-legged?
• Are both shoulders level?
• Is your body upright or do you lean to one side?

If you find you have developed running faults, see a physiotherapist who can give you special exercises to re-educate your running gait. Remember that uneven running is a common cause of overuse injury.

5

Training Log

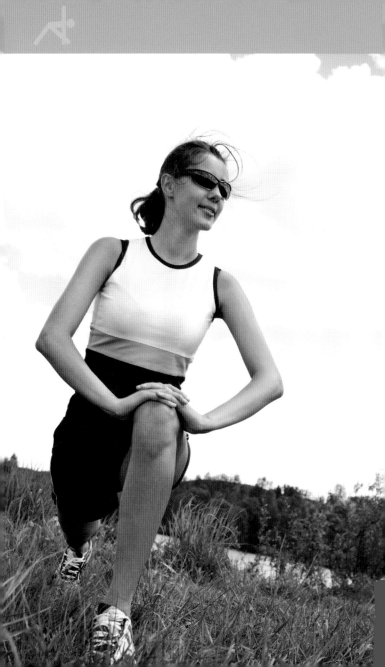

Use these charts to record your progress. Refer to page 4 for guidance.

Phase I – Beginner

No	Exercise	Average	Initial flexibility Less/ average/ more	Week 1 No of reps /sets performed	Week 1 Less/ average/ more	Week 2 No of reps /sets performed	Week 2 Less/ average/ more	Week 3 No of reps /sets performed	Week 3 Less/ average/ more
1	Hamstrings – active knee extension	Knee 20° short of fully locked							
2	Rectus femoris stretch – standing	Heel 10 cm from buttock							
3	Calf lunge	Knee mid-foot							

No	Exercise	Average	Initial flexibility	Week 1		Week 2		Week 3	
			Less/ average/ more	No of reps /sets performed	Less/ average/ more	No of reps /sets performed	Less/ average/ more	No of reps /sets performed	Less/ average/ more
4	Thoracic spine – sitting	Thoracic spine just short of straight							
5	Spinal rotation – two legs	Knee 10 cm from floor							
6	Soles of the feet	Big toe joint at 80° angle							

Phase II – Intermediate

No	Exercise	Average	Initial flexibility	Week 1		Week 2		Week 3	
			Less/ average/ more	No of reps /sets performed	Less/ average/ more	No of reps /sets performed	Less/ average/ more	No of reps /sets performed	Less/ average/ more
1	Spinal rotation – lying	Knee 10 cm from floor							
2	Lower back extension – lying	Upper chest lifted clear of floor							
3	Lower back flexion – lying	Knee 10 cm from chest							

No	Exercise	Average	Initial flexibility	Week 1		Week 2		Week 3	
			Less/ average/ more	No of reps /sets performed	Less/ average/ more	No of reps /sets performed	Less/ average/ more	No of reps /sets performed	Less/ average/ more
4	Anterior tibials	Ankle 2.5 cm from ground							
5	Hip adductors – long sitting	Knee 15 cm from ground							
6	Knee extension – with towel	Knee nearly locked							

No	Exercise	Average	Initial flexibility	Week 1		Week 2		Week 3	
			Less/ average/ more	No of reps /sets performed	Less/ average/ more	No of reps /sets performed	Less/ average/ more	No of reps /sets performed	Less/ average/ more
7	Hip flexors – Thomas test	Lower leg 10° above horizontal							
8	Iliotibial band	Upper leg 10° above horizontal							
9	Deep calf and Achilles	Knee over mid-foot							

Phase III – Advanced

No	Exercise	Average	Initial flexibility	Weeks 1/2		Weeks 2/3		Weeks 3/4	
			Less/ average/ more	No of reps /sets performed	Less/ average/ more	No of reps /sets performed	Less/ average/ more	No of reps /sets performed	Less/ average/ more
1	Hip adductors – wall support	90° angle between legs							
2	Lateral flexion – standing	Upper shoulder above groin							
3	Anterior chest and shoulders	Upper arms at 20° to body surface							

No	Exercise	Average	Initial flexibility	Weeks 1/2		Weeks 2/3		Weeks 3/4	
			Less/ average/ more	No of reps /sets performed	Less/ average/ more	No of reps /sets performed	Less/ average/ more	No of reps /sets performed	Less/ average/ more
4	Gluteals	Hip held at 80° bend							
5	Hip flexors – supine lying	Upper leg 10 cm from chest							
6	Hamstrings – lying on back	Straight leg 70° to vertical							

No	Exercise	Average	Initial flexibility	Weeks 1/2		Weeks 2/3		Weeks 3/4	
			Less/ average/ more	No of reps /sets performed	Less/ average/ more	No of reps /sets performed	Less/ average/ more	No of reps /sets performed	Less/ average/ more
7	Leg swing – forwards/backwards	Leg 45° to horizontal							
8	Leg swing – sideways	Leg 30° to horizontal							
9	Calf stretch – sprint start	Back heel 5 cm from ground							

6

Terms you should know

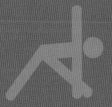

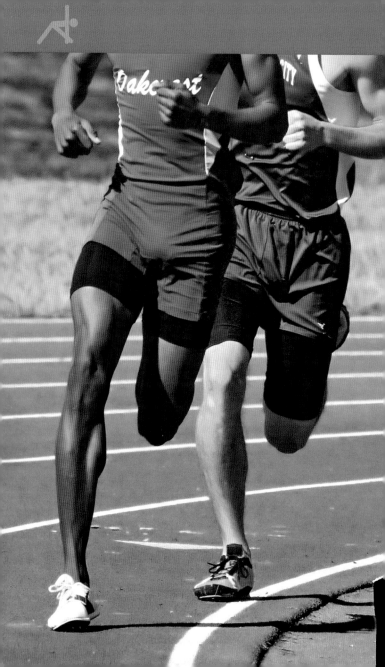

Terms you should know

abduction – moving a limb away from you

adduction – moving a limb in towards you

agility – training which combines stretch, balance and strength

arousal level – how 'psyched up' you are for exercise

cardiovascular (CV) training – working your heart/lungs/circulation using exercise that makes you out of breath

delayed onset muscle soreness (DOMS) – stiffness and soreness in muscles which occur one or two days after training

dynamic stretch – stretching while moving

extension – straightening a joint

flexion – bending a joint

general exercise – exercise which works several body parts at once

iliotibial band – a tight band of tissue travelling down the outside of your thigh

ischaemic muscle pain – 'the burn' felt during exercise, due to the build-up of muscle acids

isolation exercise – exercise that focuses on a single body part

isometric – a muscle contraction where you tense and hold

lumbar spine – your lower back

motivation – how keen you are to exercise

movement range (or **range of motion**) – the amount of movement in a joint

muscle fibre – each muscle is made up of thousands of microscopic fibres, arranged a little like the bristles on a shaving brush

muscle imbalance – when one group of muscles is unnaturally stronger or more flexible than another

overuse injury – one that comes on over time

periodisation – a method of splitting your training programme up into sections so you do not practise all exercises in each workout

plantarfascia – a bowstring of tissue supporting the arch of your foot

pronation – turning the hand or foot downwards (palm to the floor or sole of the foot to the floor)

repetition or rep – a single movement or exercise

Set – a group of repetitions, for example one set of five reps

Shin splint – pain in the muscles along the shin bones

Static stretch – stretch and hold

Thoracic spine – the upper back

Training intensity – how hard you exercise

Training volume – how much exercise (numbers of sets and reps) you do

Traumatic injury – one that occurs suddenly

Treadmill – road running machine seen in gyms

Workout – the time you spend exercising